Paleo Diet Recipes

Includes 48 Amazingly Easy Paleo Recipes

Summary

This book is compiled with some amazing paleo recipes for the health conscious. Easy to make and appetizing, this book with take to through the world of paleo goodness with simplicity and class!

Paleo is a nutritious diet that uses fruits, vegetables and lean proteins to help you lose weight. Paleo diet also uses healthy fats from olive oil and nut oil to build a complete nutritious diet plan that helps you stay fit and healthy.

Disclaimer and Terms of Use:

Effort has been made to ensure that the information in this book is accurate and complete, however, the author and the publisher do not warrant the accuracy of the information, text and graphics contained within the book due to the rapidly changing nature of science, research, known and unknown facts and internet. The Author and the publisher do not hold any responsibility for errors, omissions or contrary interpretation of the subject matter herein. This book is presented solely for motivational and informational purposes only.

Contents

Introduction

Paleo diet with all its scrumptious goodness also helps improve signs of diabetes and cardio vascular diseases, as also proven through research. When compared to the Mediterranean diet, a paleo diet has proved to be better in terms of health benefits it provides. Not only is the paleo diet used to lose weight, people following this diet have also improved lipids and reduced pain from autoimmunity.

In this book, you will find a number of options for your lunches, dinners and snacks, so you don't have to worry about the menu for the next month, at least. Sit back and enjoy the simple recipes compiled specially for you. This will provide you everything; variety, taste and health, all in one place so you do not have to worry!

Soups

Some amazing soups to appetize and delight! Try some of these easy paleo recipes to excite your taste buds and lose weight!

Cantaloupe Soup

Serves Two

Ingredients:

- 4 cups cubed ripe cantaloupe

- One and one-half cups ripe strawberries, hulled

- 1 cup fresh apple juice

- One-half cup dry white wine

- 2 tablespoons fresh lime juice

- 1 teaspoon finely chopped fresh ginger

- 2 tablespoons snipped fresh mint

- Sliced strawberries and mint leaves (optional)

Instructions:

1. Blend all the ingredients in a food processor until all the ingredients reach the same consistency.

2. Refrigerate for four hours.

3. Serve.

Mutton Soup

Serves Six to Eight

Ingredients:

1 meat bone

A couple pounds of mutton or beef soup meat

5 quarts water

Vegetables

Salt to taste

Black pepper to taste

Small piece of garlic

Instructions:

1. Boil all the ingredients in a pot on medium heat until the broth reduces by one to two cups.

2. Discard the bone.

3. Thicken the soup with a mixture of cornstarch and water.

4. Serve.

Vegetable Soup

Serves Four

Ingredients:

- 1 1/2 cups onions, chopped

- 4 medium carrots, sliced

- 3 celery ribs, sliced

- 1/2 teaspoon salt

- 1/2 teaspoon pepper

- 1/4 cup all-purpose flour

- 1/2 cup water

- 1 cup cabbage, chopped

- 2 tablespoons olive oil

- 3 cups vegetable broth

- 4 medium potatoes, peeled and sliced

- 4 medium tomatoes, chopped

- 2 garlic cloves, minced

Instructions:

1. Boil all the ingredients in a pot on medium heat until the broth reduces by one to two cups.

2. Thicken the soup with a mixture of cornstarch and water.

3. Serve.

Dumplings in a Soup of Your Choice

Serves Four

Ingredients:

2 1/4 to 1/2 cups reduced-fat biscuit/baking mix, paleo-friendly

1 tablespoon fresh parsley, minced

Up to 1 cup cold water

1 cup carrots, shredded

5 cups of soup/broth (your choice)

Instructions:

1. Mix all ingredients in a bowl until you have a consistent mixture.

2. Shape the dumplings into a ball or any other shape you like.

3. Boil the soup/broth then drop dumpling balls into broth.

4. Let it simmer for 15 minutes.

5. Serve.

Celery Soup

Serves Six to Eight

Here is how to make amazing paleo recipes at home:

Ingredients:

1 cup onions, small diced

1/2 cup celery, small diced

1 ham hock (1 1/4 pounds), skin scored

10 cups chicken stock (or canned low sodium chicken broth)

2 teaspoons salt

1 1/2 teaspoons coarsely ground black pepper

1/2 cup red bell pepper, small diced

1 tablespoon plus 1 teaspoon garlic, minced

Instructions:

1. Boil all the ingredients in a pot on medium heat until the broth reduces by one to two cups.

2. Thicken the soup with a mixture of cornstarch and water.

3. Serve.

Garden Vegetable Soup

Serves Four to Six

Ingredients:

6 sprigs parsley

2 bay leaves

2 tablespoons olive oil or butter

2 cups broccoli or cauliflower florets cut into bite-size pieces

1 cup diced zucchini (large dice)

1 cup diced yellow squash (large dice)

One 10-ounce bag prewashed spinach

2 cups diced onions

1 1/2 cups diced carrots

1 1/2 cups diced celery (small dice, with or without leaves)

2 tablespoons minced garlic

8 ounces button mushrooms, wiped clean, stemmed, and quartered (about 2 cups)

4 quarts vegetable broth

1 1/2 teaspoons salt

Instructions:

1. Boil all the ingredients in a pot on medium heat until the broth reduces by one to two cups.

2. Thicken the soup with a mixture of cornstarch and water.

3. Serve.

Green Veggie Soup

Serves Two

Ingredients:

- 2 cups raw broccoli

- 4 cups low-sodium vegetable broth

- Salt and pepper, to taste

- 1 head kale stems removed

- 1 bag spinach

- 2 garlic cloves, minced

Instructions:

1. Boil all the ingredients in a pot on medium heat until the broth reduces by one to two cups.

2. Thicken the soup with a mixture of cornstarch and water.

3. Serve.

Garden Harvest Soup

Serves Four to Six

Ingredients:

- 1 tablespoon olive oil

- 1 medium onion, chopped

- 1 carrot, chopped

- 4 garlic cloves, thinly sliced

- 2 cups water

- 1 small head cabbage, thinly sliced

- 1 red bell pepper, chopped

- 2 quarts (8 cups) low-salt vegetable or chicken stock or broth

- 1 can (28 ounces) whole, crushed or diced tomatoes, un-drained

- Optional garnishes: chopped fresh parsley, chopped fresh cilantro

Instructions:

1. Boil all the ingredients in a pot on medium heat until the broth reduces by one to two cups.

2. Thicken the soup with a mixture of cornstarch and water.

3. Garnish and serve.

Beef Mole Chili

Serves Four

Ingredients:

3 tablespoons olive oil

2 1/2 pounds ground beef

8 medium yellow onions, sliced thin

1 head of garlic (about 10 cloves), minced

4 1/2 teaspoons ground cumin

4 1/2 teaspoons ground coriander

Freshly ground black pepper

8 scallions (green parts only), chopped

1 bunch cilantro, minced

2/3 cup espresso powder

5 ounces unsweetened chocolate, roughly chopped

1 tablespoon salt, plus more to taste

4 2-5 ounce dark chocolate bars (70% or higher cocoa content)

4 1/2 teaspoons dried oregano

2 1/2 teaspoons chili powder

4 28-ounce cans crushed tomatoes, with their juice

1 quart chicken broth or beef broth

2 cinnamon sticks

Instructions:

1. Boil all the ingredients in a pot on medium heat until the broth reduces by one to two cups. Discard the cinnamon sticks.

2. Thicken the soup with a mixture of cornstarch and water.

3. Serve.

Broccoli and Rosemary Soup Delight

Serves Four to Six

Ingredients:

2 tablespoons olive oil

2 cups small-diced onion

1 cup small-diced celery

1 cup small-diced red bell pepper

1 tablespoon plus 1 teaspoon salt

1/2 teaspoon freshly ground black pepper

2 tablespoons minced garlic

1 bay leaf

4 cups water

1 1/2 pounds broccoli, tough stem ends trimmed, chopped into bite- sized pieces

1 sprig fresh rosemary

Grated zest of 1 lemon

2 teaspoons freshly squeezed lemon juice

Extra-virgin olive oil, for drizzling

1 teaspoon dried Italian herbs

1/4 teaspoon crushed red pepper

8 cups chicken stock or canned low-sodium chicken broth

Instructions:

1. Boil all the ingredients in a pot over medium heat for thirty minutes.

2. Thicken the soup with a mixture of cornstarch and water.

3. Serve.

Tuscan Style Soup

Serves Three to Four

Ingredients:

- 1 1/4 cup eggplant, peeled and cubed

- 1 cup water

- 1/2 tsp Italian seasoning, dried

- 12 oz. can chicken broth, reduced sodium

- 1 can of whole tomatoes, no salt added, un-drained and chopped (14 1/2-ounce)

- 1 can sliced mushrooms, drained (OR 1 cup fresh mushrooms, sliced)

- 1 clove garlic, minced

- 1 small summer (yellow) squash, coarsely chopped

- 1/4 tsp salt

- 1/8 tsp pepper

Instructions:

1. Boil all the ingredients in a pot over medium heat for thirty minutes.

2. Thicken the soup with a mixture of cornstarch and water.

3. Serve.

Leek Soup

Serves Three to Four

Ingredients:

- 1 large or 2 small leeks (about 1 pound)

- 2 bay leaves

- 20 black peppercorns

- 5 cups chicken stock or canned, low-sodium chicken broth

- 11/2 teaspoons salt

- 3/4 teaspoon freshly ground white pepper

- 2 tablespoons snipped fresh chives

- 4 sprigs fresh thyme

- 2 tablespoons olive oil

- 2 slices bacon, diced

- 1/2 cup dry white wine

Instructions:

1. Boil all the ingredients in a pot over medium heat until the broth reduces by one to two cups.

2. Thicken the soup with a mixture of cornstarch and water.
3. Serve.

Broccoli Soup

Serves Three to Four

Ingredients:

2 tablespoons olive oil

1 1/2 cups thinly sliced yellow onions

1 tablespoon sliced garlic

5 cups chicken stock or canned, low-sodium chicken broth

4 cups broccoli florets

Simple Croutons, for garnish (optional)

1 teaspoon salt

1/4 teaspoon cayenne pepper

Instructions:

1. Boil all the ingredients in a pot over medium heat until the broth reduces by one to two cups.

2. Thicken the soup with a mixture of cornstarch and water.

3. Serve.

Chicken and Celery Soup

Serves Three to Four

Ingredients:

2 pounds boneless, skinless chicken breasts, cut into 3/4-inch dice

1 tablespoon Emeril's Original Essence or Creole Seasoning

1 tablespoon olive oil

1 teaspoon dried basil

1 teaspoon salt

1/4 teaspoon crushed red pepper

2 quarts chicken stock or canned, low-sodium chicken broth, plus more if needed

One 5-ounce bag prewashed spinach

2 cups diced onions (small dice)

1 1/2 cups diced carrots (small dice)

1 1/2 cups diced celery (small dice)

1 tablespoon minced garlic

Instructions:

1. Boil all the ingredients in a pot over medium heat until the broth reduces by one to two cups.

2. Thicken the soup with a mixture of cornstarch and water.

3. Serve.

Cure-All Chicken Soup

Serves Three to Four

Ingredients:

Salt, for cooking the rice

2/3 pound chicken breast halves, fresh or frozen (skinless, boneless)

1 cup long-grain rice

3 medium-size ribs of celery (for about 1 1/2 cups diced)

1 clove fresh garlic, minced (or 1 teaspoon bottled minced garlic)

1 teaspoon fresh ginger, finely minced (or bottled minced ginger)

2 cans fat-free chicken broth (or 4 cups homemade chicken stock), about 14 ounces each)

1/4 teaspoon black pepper, or to taste

2 teaspoons olive oil

1 large onion (for about 1 cup chopped)

2 medium-size carrots (for about 1 cup chopped)

Instructions:

1. Boil all the ingredients in a pot over medium heat until the broth reduces by one to two cups.

2. Thicken the soup with a mixture of cornstarch and water.

3. Serve.

Egg and Lemon Soup

Serves Three to Four

Ingredients:

  5 cups chicken broth

  1 Onion (quartered)

  Juice from 3 to 5 Lemons

  1/4 teaspoon Cornstarch (add at the end)

  1 Carrot (thickly sliced)

  1 Head of Garlic (halved crosswise)

  4 sprigs Fresh Thyme

  1 tablespoon Kosher Salt

  1 Bay Leaf

  1 tablespoon Black Peppercorns

  3 to 5 Eggs (add at the end)

Instructions:

1. Boil all the ingredients in a pot over medium heat until the broth reduces by one to two cups.

2. Thicken the soup with a mixture of cornstarch and water.

3. Add lightly beaten eggs.

4. Serve.

Roasted Pumpkin Soup

Serves Five to Six

Ingredients:

4 pounds sugar or pie pumpkin or other winter
squash, such as butternut or acorn, peeled,
seeded, and cut into 3-inch chunks

1/4 cup olive oil

1 tablespoon salt

1 teaspoon freshly ground black or white pepper

4 cups water

2 ounces (about 2 bunches) fresh chives, snipped
to 3-inch lengths (2 cups), basil leaves, or mint
leaves

3/4 cup olive oil

1/8 teaspoon salt

3 cups chopped onions

1/2 cup chopped carrots

1 clove garlic, smashed

1 or 2 sprigs fresh thyme

1 cup brandy

4 cups chicken stock or canned low-sodium
chicken broth

Herb Oil of choice, for garnish

Instructions:

1. Preheat oven to 350 F (175 C).

2. In a pot add olive oil and caramelize the squash on medium heat.

3. Add rest of the ingredients.

4. Boil all the ingredients until the broth reduces by one to two cups.

5. Thicken the soup with a mixture of cornstarch and water.

6. Transfer the broth to a casserole and bake in a casserole for 15 minutes.

7. Serve with herb oil on top.

Zucchini Tomato Soup

Serves One to Two

Ingredients:

2 small zucchini, coarsely chopped

1/4 cup chopped red onion

1 small tomato, cut into thin wedges

Dash each pepper and dried basil

2 tablespoons shredded cheddar cheese, optional

1 to 2 tablespoons crumbled cooked bacon, optional

1 1/2 teaspoons Light Olive Oil

1/8 teaspoon salt

1 cup spicy hot V8 juice

Instructions:

1. In a pot, boil all the ingredients for 30 minutes.

2. Thicken the soup with a mixture of corn flour and water.

3. Serve.

Tomato and Corn Soup with Basil

Serves Two

Ingredients:

- 1 cup fresh or thawed frozen corn kernels

- 2 large tomatoes, seeded and chopped

- 1 cup water

- 3 tablespoons fresh lime juice

- Sea salt, plus more for sprinkling

- Pinch of freshly ground black pepper, plus more for sprinkling

- 1 teaspoon grated lime zest

- 1 cup finely chopped fresh basil, plus basil leaves for garnish

- 2 tablespoons cold- pressed extra-virgin olive oil, plus more for drizzling

- 1 garlic clove

Instructions:

4. In a pot boil all the ingredients for thirty minutes.

5. Thicken the soup with some corn flour and water mixtures.

6.   Serve.

Tomato Sweet potato Bisque

Serves Two

Ingredients:

2 tablespoons extra virgin olive oil

2 medium carrots, coarsely chopped

1 jalapeno chilies, stemmed, seeded, and chopped

4 garlic cloves, chopped

2 sprigs fresh thyme

4 fresh basil leaves

1 celery rib, coarsely chopped

1 jumbo sweet onion, coarsely chopped

Kosher salt

One 14.5-ouncecan diced fire-roasted tomatoes

1 Quart Vegetable Stock

1 medium sweet potato, peeled and chopped

1 cup paleo mayo (at the end)

Freshly ground black pepper

Instructions:

1. In a large pot, add some olive oil and let it warm over medium heat. Turn to high heat and add the rest of the ingredients.

1. Include the broth.

2. Let the broth simmer on low heat for thirty minutes.

3. Transfer to a blender.

4. Blend until a nice mixture is formed.

5. Serve.

Appetizers and Salads

Some amazing appetizers and salads are compiled especially for you to enjoy your weight loss regimen, without depriving your taste buds!

Lagasse

Serves Two

Ingredients:

1/4 cup low-sodium soy sauce

1/4 cup dry sherry

3 tablespoons canned low- sodium vegetable, chicken, or beef broth

1 teaspoon toasted sesame oil

1 teaspoon cornstarch

1 teaspoon raw honey

3 small carrots, halved lengthwise and cut into 1/8-inch-thick half-moons on the diagonal (about 1 1/2 cups)

1 celery stalk, thinly sliced on the diagonal (about 1/2 cup)

2 cups halved broccoli florets

2 cups sliced shiitake mushrooms (about 4 ounces)

2 cups 1/4-inch sliced red cabbage

1 cup snow peas, ends trimmed (about 4 ounces)

1 cup bean sprouts

3 tablespoons olive oil

1 1/2 tablespoons peeled and minced fresh ginger

1 1/2 tablespoons minced garlic

1 bunch green onions, cut into 2-inch pieces on the diagonal (about 1 cup)

2 to 3 small dried hot red chilies

1/2 green bell pepper, cut into 1-inch dice (about 3/4 cup)

1/2 red bell pepper, cut into 1-inch dice (about 3/4 cup)

Steamed jasmine or other rice, for serving

Instructions:

1. In a large pot, add some olive oil and let it warm.

6. Add the ingredients one by one to the oil.

7. Cook for ten minutes over high heat.

8. Serve with steamed rice.

BBQ Chicken Strips

Serves Two

Ingredients:

> 1 3-pound Chicken (cut into 8 pieces) cut into thin strips
>
> Salt and Freshly Ground Pepper
>
> Extra Virgin Olive Oil
>
> BBQ sauce
>
> 2 tablespoons chicken rub

Instructions:

2. Marinate the chicken for one to two hours in all the ingredients.

3. In a skillet, add some olive oil on medium heat.

4. Cook the chicken in olive oil for fifteen minutes over low heat, seven to eight minutes on each side.

Grilled Chicken Strips recipe with Mustard BBQ Sauce

Serves Two

Ingredients:

6-7 good sized fresh blueberries

2 pounds chicken breasts, lightly pounded and cut into thin strips

2 ounces plain vodka

2 ounces of blueberry flavored vodka

1 teaspoon of low carb sugar syrup (see recipe above)

1 Tablespoon BBQ sauce

1 Tablespoon mustard sauce

Instructions:

1. Marinate the chicken for one to two hours in all the ingredients.

2. In a skillet add some olive oil and let it warm.

3. Cook the chicken in olive oil for fifteen minutes over low heat, seven to eight minutes on each side.

Sweet and Gold Potato Salad

Serves Two

Ingredients:

1 lb. Yukon gold potatoes, peeled and cut into a 3/4-inch dice

1 lb. red sweet potatoes, peeled and cut into a 3/4-inch dice

Kosher salt and freshly ground pepper

4 large eggs

1 C Paleo Mayo

1/2 tsp. cayenne pepper

2 celery ribs with leaves, minced (3/4 C)

3 scallions, trimmed and finely chipped

1/2 C sweet relish

1 tsp. Dijon mustard

1/4 C chopped mixed fresh herbs

Instructions:

1. Boil the eggs and potatoes. You want the eggs hardboiled and the potatoes done.

2. Cube the ingredients and place in a large bowl.

3. Add in the rest of the ingredients.

4. Toss and serve.

Lemon Dill Potato Salad

Serves Two

Ingredients:

3 pounds red bliss potato, cut into 1/2" cubes and boiled

1 cup paleo mayo

1 tablespoon red wine vinegar

1/4 cup fresh dill, chopped

Salt and pepper

2 lemons, zest and juice

Instructions:

1. Cube the ingredients and place in a large bowl.

2. Add in the rest of the ingredients.

3. Serve.

**Paleo Mayonnaise

1 egg

1 cup of Olive oil

Juice of half a lemon or lime

Salt to taste

1. Combine all of the ingredients in a jar. Let the egg yolk sink to the bottom of the jar.
2. Use an immersion stick blender for 10-20 seconds or until you have a smooth paste.
3. Add in the salt.
4. Other ingredients such as garlic, Dijon powder, black pepper etc can be used to give your mayo more taste.

Apple Compote Napoleon

Serves Two

Ingredients:

2 tablespoon olive oil

4 granny smith apples, peeled and diced

1 teaspoon cinnamon

1/2 cup golden raisins

1 cup toasted walnuts, roughly chopped

caramel sauce

Salt to taste

2 tablespoons lemon juice

3 tablespoons cornstarch

1 teaspoon vanilla extract

¼ cup raw honey

Instructions:

1. Cube the ingredients and place in a large bowl.

2. Add in the rest of the ingredients.

3. Toss and serve.

Spiced Ginger Cider

Serves five to six

Ingredients:

- 32 ounces unfiltered apple cider

- 2 cinnamon sticks

- 2 ginger tea bags

Instructions:

1. Heat the cider on medium heat over a stove. Turn off the heat.

2. Add cinnamon sticks to the cider. Take out the sticks after a minute.

3. Add tea bags.

4. You are done. Serve!

Strawberry Watermelon Parfait

Parfait for Two

Ingredients:

- 1 pint raspberries

- 4 crispy basil leaves

- 1 tablespoon lemon zest, finely grated

- 2 teaspoons fresh lemon juice

- 4 large basil leaves

- 1 teaspoon Olive oil

- 1 tablespoon lemon juice (reserve zest and remaining juice for cream)

- 1 small watermelon, about 3 cups

- 1 pint strawberries, hulled and quartered

- 2 cups sponge cake, 1" cubes (For serving)

Instructions:

1. Add in all the ingredients in a blender and blend.

2. Serve the mixture over sponge cake in a cocktail glass.

Lemon Rosemary Chicken

This chicken recipe is enough for two.

Ingredients:

2 pounds chicken breasts, lightly pounded and cut into 1 inch chunks

4 lemons, juiced

Freshly ground black pepper

2 large white onions, cut into 1 1/2 inch chunks

3 garlic cloves, minced

1 tablespoon ground rosemary

Instructions:

1. Add all the ingredients to the chicken and marinate the chicken for half an hour.

2. In a skillet, add some olive oil and cook the chicken for ten minutes on each side.

3. Serve.

Chicken Caesar Salad

Serves Two

Ingredients:

- 1/2 cup plain Greek Yogurt

- 1 teaspoon olive oil

- 1/2 lemon, juiced

- 2 medium garlic cloves, minced

- 1/2 teaspoon balsamic vinegar

- 1 tablespoon Worcestershire sauce

- 1 teaspoon freshly ground black pepper

- 1 head romaine lettuce, chilled and sliced

- 1 1/2 teaspoons red wine vinegar

- 2 teaspoons Dijon mustard

- 1 tablespoon anchovy paste

Instructions:

1. Add in all the ingredients in a salad bowl.

2. Toss and serve.

Root Vegetable Ragout

Serves Two to Three

Ingredients:

- 2 medium carrots

- 2 medium parsnips

- 1 small rutabaga

- 1 tablespoon olive oil

- 3 cup chicken Stock

- 1 medium turnip

- 1 medium Yukon gold potato

- Freshly ground black pepper

- 2 tablespoons fresh flat-leaf parsley leaves, chopped

- 2 tablespoons fresh thyme leaves, chopped

- Freshly grated zest of 1 lemon

- Kosher salt

- 1 small yellow onion, cut

Instructions:

1. Dice all the vegetables.

2. In a skillet, add the butter, followed by the onion. Stir for two minutes and let the onions soften. Add in all the vegetables.

3. Cook for ten minutes after adding all the ingredients. Stir fry for ten minutes before including the stock.

4. Let the stock simmer on low heat for twenty minutes Add the thyme, parsley and lemon zest. Taste and add salt and pepper as needed.

5. Serve.

Charred Corn Salad

Serves One to Two

Ingredients:

4 ears corn, cut off the cob

4 teaspoons olive oil

1 tablespoon sherry vinegary

Salt and freshly ground black pepper

1 red onion, sliced

1 tablespoon slivered green olives

2 scallions, white and tender green parts, thinly sliced

1 tablespoon chopped fresh basil

Instructions:

1. Add in all the ingredients in a bowl.

2. Serve.

Summer Corn Salad

Serves One to Two

Ingredients:

4 ears fresh corn

1/2 small red onion, thinly sliced

¼ cup paleo cheddar cheese

1/2 lime, juiced

1/2 teaspoon ground cumin

1/4 teaspoon cayenne pepper, or to taste

2 tablespoons olive oil

Salt and freshly ground black pepper

1 (3-ounce) bunch cilantro, leaves only

2 heads Belgian endive

Instructions:

1. Add in all the ingredients in a bowl.

2. Toss and serve.

Stir- fry Green Beans

Serves Two to Three

Ingredients:

- 2 pounds salmon fillets

- 4 tbsp. sesame oil

- 1/2 cup tamari soy sauce

- 1 teaspoon minced garlic

- 1/2 teaspoon ground ginger

- 1/2 teaspoon basil

- 1 teaspoon oregano leaves

- 1/4 teaspoon thyme

- 1/2 teaspoon rosemary

- 1/4 teaspoon tarragon

- 1/2 cup chopped fresh mushrooms

- 1/2 cup chopped green onions

Instructions:

1. Preheat oven to 350 F(175 C)

2. Marinate the salmon with all the mentioned ingredients.

3. Bake for 10 minutes.

Sweet Stir Prize

Serves One

Ingredients:

2 Tbsp. low-sodium soy sauce

1/2 Tbsp. Sriracha or other Asian-style chili sauce

2 Tbsp. orange juice

1 medium sweet potato, half done, peeled and sliced into thin rounds

4 cups broccoli florets

1 small yellow onion, sliced

2 cloves chopped garlic

1 Tbsp. fresh minced ginger

1 Tbsp. rice wine vinegar

1/2 Tbsp. cornstarch

1 tbsp. Olive Oil

1 lb. boneless skinless chicken thighs cut into bite-size pieces

Instructions:

1. In a skillet, add the oil and let it warm on medium heat before you add the onions and ginger. Next, add the chicken and stir for two minutes.

2. Next, add the sweet potatoes and broccoli with all the sauces and the orange juice.

3. Stir fry all the ingredients together for around five minutes. To thicken the sauce, use corn flour and water mixture.

4. Plate.

5. You are done.

Mint and WatermelonSalad

Serves One

Ingredients:

1 Small to medium sized watermelon (approx. 4lbs), diced into cubes

16 oz. non-dairy cheese

1 Small bunch of mint

2 Splashes of red wine vinegar

4 T. Extra virgin olive oil

Sea salt

Instructions:

1. Transfer the ingredients to a salad bowl.

2. Add in salt and olive oil.

3. Toss and serve.

Chilled Watermelon Slices with Lime

Serves Two

Ingredients:

  1 watermelon, chilled and sliced

  1/4 cup raw honey

  1/2 cup mint, chopped

  1/2 cup fresh lime juice

  Zest from one lime

Instructions:

  1. Plate and dress.

  2. Serve.

Marinated Olives

Serves Six to Eight

Ingredients:

2 cups Alfonso Olives

2 Tablespoon chopped fresh rosemary (bruise)

2 cloves garlic thinly sliced

1/4 cup red wine vinegar

zest of 1 lemon

1 teaspoon red chili flakes

Instructions:

1. Marinate the olives overnight in the refrigerator.

2. You are ready to serve! Serve it with any main course or snack of your choice; it will go best with baked fish/ chicken items.

Watermelon Tomato Salad

Serves Two

Ingredients:

- 1 mini seedless watermelon, about 4 pounds

- 1 3/4 pounds heirloom tomatoes, sliced

- 2 Tablespoons lemon juice

- 2 Persian cucumbers, sliced

- 2 Tablespoons extra-virgin olive oil

- 3 oz. non-dairy cheese

- 1/2 cup fresh mint leaves

- Salt and Pepper

Instructions:

1. Plate the ingredients.

2. Toss and serve.

Bourbon Mash

Serves Four

Ingredients:

   8 large garnet sweet potatoes, boiled

   1 pint heavy cream

   3 dashes Tabasco sauce

   1 teaspoon sea salt

   1 nutmeg, freshly grated, optional

   3/4 cup bourbon

   1/2 cup molasses

Instructions:

   1. Blend the ingredients in a food processor.

   2. Serve.

Drinks

For those hot and sunny days, these paleo drinks will help you enjoy the beauty of the sunny summers while shedding those extra pounds!

Berry Pink Lemonade

Serves One

Ingredients:

1 cup lemon juice, freshly squeezed or bottled

5 cups water

1 Lemon (optional, for slices)

1 cup strawberries, sliced

Instructions:

1. Add in all the ingredients in a blender and blend.

2. Serve with ice.

Royal Punch

Serves One

Ingredients:

2 parts Beefeater London Dry Gin

2 parts fresh lemonade (American style)

Angostura bitters to taste

1 part Dubonnet

1 part pomegranate juice

Instructions:

1. Add in all the ingredients in a blender and blend.

2. Serve with ice in a cocktail glass.

Shamrock Punch

Serves One

Ingredients:

14oz. Bombay Sapphire gin

6 oz. Lemon juice

Black peppercorn

7 oz. St-Germaine artisanal French elderflower liqueur

1 spring of sage

6 oz. Fresh guava juice

Instructions:

1. Add in all the ingredients in a blender and blend.

2. Serve in a cocktail glass with ice.

Mint Sprigs Punch

Serves One

Ingredients:

  8-10 mint sprigs

  4 liters plain seltzer water

  1 12-cup muffin tin (silicone is best)

  2 liters store-bought lemonade (Our favorite brand is Newman's Own Virgin Lemonade)

Instructions:

1. Add all of the ingredients in a blender and blend.

4. Serve in a cocktail glass with ice.

Tangerine Pomegranate Punch

Serves One

Ingredients:

1 cup fresh tangerine juice

3 tbsp. honey

Pomegranate seeds, to garnish

1/2 cup pomegranate juice

Crushed ice

Instructions:

1. Add all of the ingredients in a blender and blend until smooth.

2. Serve.

Green Tea Water Melon Super Punch

Serves two

Ingredients:

2 cups ice

4 cups cubed seedless watermelon

1 cup chopped fresh pineapple

1/4 cup agave nectar

2 teaspoons unsweetened matcha green tea powder

1 cup nonfat Greek yogurt, such as 0% Fage Total

1/4 fresh lime juice

Crushed ice

Instructions:

1. Add all of the ingredients in a blender and blend until smooth.

2. Serve.

Strawberry Lemonade

Serves two

Ingredients:

> 3 cups water
>
> 4 cups chopped fresh strawberry
>
> ½ cup maple syrup
>
> 2 3 inch strips lemon zest
>
> 3 sprigs fresh basil
>
> 1 cup fresh lemon juice
>
> 2 cups sparkling water
>
> 6 ounces gin
>
> Crushed ice

Instructions:

1. Add all of the ingredients in a blender and blend until smooth.
2. Serve.

Strawberry Basil Soda

Serves two

Ingredients:

- 1 pound Strawberries (trimmed)

- 2 tablespoons Lemon Juice

- 2 tablespoons of raw honey

- Some salt to rim the glasses

- Seltzer

- Juice and Zest of 1 Lime (plus the zest of another lime for rimming glass)

- 1/2 cup Basil Leaves (plus 5 more for rimming glass)

- Crushed ice

Instructions:

1. Add all of the ingredients in a blender and blend until smooth.

2. Serve.

Conclusion

Like you must have read, this book is especially designed for individuals who want to follow easy and healthy recipes.

It has been made sure that the ingredients used in the recipes are simple and the recipes are easy are understand. As you have seen, there is no extensive preparation required to prepare your paleo goodness, they are made easily with a few simple steps.

From breakfast to dinner and snack, this book is complete. You can find a wide variety of recipes all in one book, so you do not have to worry at all!

What are you waiting for? Avail the health benefits following these simple recipes and enjoy the goodness of some amazing healthy foods.

As you have seen, the steps are simple, so you don't have to spend hours preparing some deliciousness for yourself and your family. So get going!

Good luck!